EASY KETO DIET RECIPES 2021

DELICIOUS KETO RECIPES TO LOSE WEIGHT FOR BEGINNERS

TONY GERE

Table of Contents

Introduction

Do you want to make a change in your life? Do you want to become a healthier person who can enjoy a new and improved life? Then, you are definitely in the right place. You are about to discover a wonderful and very healthy diet that has changed millions of lives. We are talking about the Ketogenic diet, a lifestyle that will mesmerize you and that will make you a new person in no time. So, let's sit back, relax and find out more about the Ketogenic diet.

A keto diet is a low carb one. This is the first and one of the most important things you should now. During such a diet, your body makes ketones in your liver and these are used as energy.
Your body will produce less insulin and glucose and a state of ketosis is induced.
Ketosis is a natural process that appears when our food intake is lower than usual. The body will soon adapt to this state and therefore you will be able to lose weight in no time but you will also become healthier and your physical and mental performances will improve.
Your blood sugar levels will improve and you won't be predisposed to diabetes.

Also, epilepsy and heart diseases can be prevented if you are on a Ketogenic diet.

Your cholesterol will improve and you will feel amazing in no time. How does that sound?

A Ketogenic diet is simple and easy to follow as long as you follow some simple rules. You don't need to make huge changes but there are some things you should know.

So, here goes!

Now let's start our magical culinary journey!

Ketogenic lifestyle...here we come!

Enjoy!

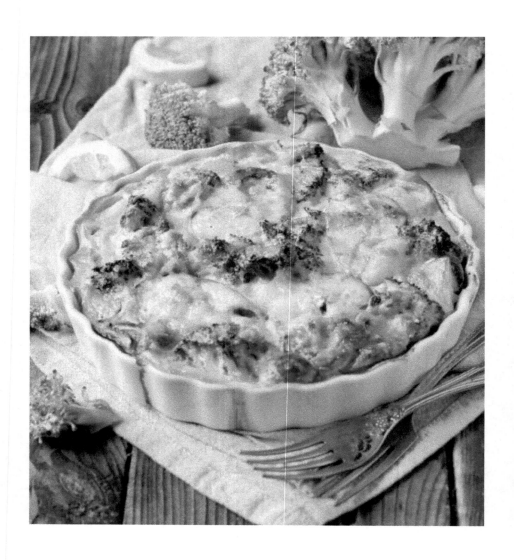

Nutrition: calories 150, fat 4, fiber 0.4, carbs 1.1, protein 3

Taco Cups

These taco cups make the perfect party appetizer!

Preparation time: 10 minutes

Cooking time: 40 minutes

Servings: 30

Ingredients:

- 1 pound beef, ground
- 2 cups cheddar cheese, shredded
- ¼ cup water
- Salt and black pepper to the taste
- 2 tablespoons cumin
- 2 tablespoons chili powder
- Pico de gallo for serving

Directions:

1. Divide spoonful of parmesan on a lined baking sheet, introduce in the oven at 350 degrees F and bake for 7 minutes.
2. Leave cheese to cool down for 1 minute, transfer them to mini cupcake molds and shape them into cups.

3. Meanwhile, heat up a pan over medium high heat, add beef, stir and cook until it browns.
4. Add the water, salt, pepper, cumin and chili powder, stir and cook for 5 minutes more.
5. Divide into cheese cups, top with pico de gallo, transfer them all to a platter and serve.

Enjoy!

Nutrition: calories 140, fat 6, fiber 0, carbs 6, protein 15

Tasty Chicken Egg Rolls

These are just what you need! It's the best keto party appetizer!

Preparation time: 2 hours and 10 minutes

Cooking time: 15 minutes

Servings: 12

Ingredients:

- 4 ounces blue cheese
- 2 cups chicken, cooked and finely chopped
- Salt and black pepper to the taste
- 2 green onions, chopped
- 2 celery stalks, finely chopped
- ½ cup tomato sauce
- ½ teaspoon erythritol
- 12 egg roll wrappers
- Vegetable oil

Directions:

1. In a bowl, mix chicken meat with blue cheese, salt, pepper, green onions, celery, tomato sauce and sweetener, stir well and keep in the fridge for 2 hours.

2. Place egg wrappers on a working surface, divide chicken mix on them, roll and seal edges.
3. Heat up a pan with vegetable oil over medium high heat, add egg rolls, cook until they are golden, flip and cook on the other side as well.
4. Arrange on a platter and serve them.

Enjoy!

Nutrition: calories 220, fat 7, fiber 2, carbs 6, protein 10

Halloumi Cheese Fries

These are so crunchy and delightful!

Preparation time: 10 minutes

Cooking time: 5 minutes

Servings: 4

Ingredients:

- 1 cup marinara sauce
- 8 ounces halloumi cheese, pat dried and sliced into fries
- 2 ounces tallow

Directions:

1. Heat up a pan with the tallow over medium high heat.
2. Add halloumi pieces, cover, cook for 2 minutes on each side and transfer to paper towels.
3. Drain excess grease, transfer them to a bowl and serve with marinara sauce on the side.

Enjoy!

Nutrition: calories 200, fat 16, fiber 1, carbs 1, protein 13

Jalapeno Crisps

These are so easy to make at home!

Preparation time: 10 minutes

Cooking time: 25 minutes

Servings: 20

Ingredients:

- 3 tablespoons olive oil
- 5 jalapenos, sliced
- 8 ounces parmesan cheese, grated
- ½ teaspoon onion powder
- Salt and black pepper to the taste
- Tabasco sauce for serving

Directions:

1. In a bowl, mix jalapeno slices with salt, pepper, oil and onion powder, toss to coat and spread on a lined baking sheet.
2. Introduce in the oven at 450 degrees F and bake for 15 minutes.
3. Take jalapeno slices out of the oven, leave them to cool down.

4. In a bowl, mix pepper slices with the cheese and press well.
5. Arrange all slices on an another lined baking sheet, introduce in the oven again and bake for 10 minutes more.
6. Leave jalapenos to cool down, arrange on a plate and serve with Tabasco sauce on the side.

Enjoy!

Nutrition: calories 50, fat 3, fiber 0.1, carbs 0.3, protein 2

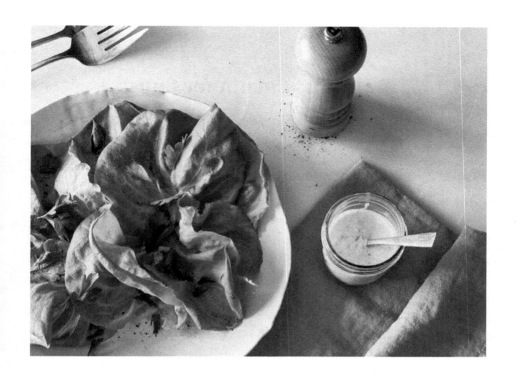

Delicious Cucumber Cups

Get ready to taste something really elegant and delicious!

Preparation time: 10 minutes

Cooking time: 0 minutes

Servings: 24

Ingredients:

- 2 cucumbers, peeled, cut into ¾ inch slices and some of the seeds scooped out
- ½ cup sour cream
- Salt and white pepper to the taste
- 6 ounces smoked salmon, flaked
- 1/3 cup cilantro, chopped
- 2 teaspoons lime juice
- 1 tablespoon lime zest
- A pinch of cayenne pepper

Directions:

1. In a bowl mix salmon with salt, pepper, cayenne, sour cream, lime juice and zest and cilantro and stir well.
2. Fill each cucumber cup with this salmon mix, arrange on a platter and serve as a keto appetizer.

Enjoy!

Nutrition: calories 30, fat 11, fiber 1, carbs 1, protein 2

Caviar Salad

This is so elegant! It's so delicious and sophisticated!

Preparation time: 6 minutes

Cooking time: 0 minutes

Servings: 16

Ingredients:

- 8 eggs, hard-boiled, peeled and mashed with a fork
- 4 ounces black caviar
- 4 ounces red caviar
- Salt and black pepper to the taste
- 1 yellow onion, finely chopped
- ¾ cup mayonnaise
- Some toast baguette slices for serving

Directions:

1. In a bowl, mix mashed eggs with mayo, salt, pepper and onion and stir well.
2. Spread eggs salad on toasted baguette slices, and top each with caviar.

Enjoy!

Nutrition: calories 122, fat 8, fiber 1, carbs 4, protein 7

Marinated Kebabs

This is the perfect appetizer for a summer barbecue!

Preparation time: 20 minutes

Cooking time: 10 minutes

Servings: 6

Ingredients:

- 1 red bell pepper, cut into chunks
- 1 green bell pepper, cut into chunks
- 1 orange bell pepper, cut into chunks
- 2 pounds sirloin steak, cut into medium cubes
- 4 garlic cloves, minced
- 1 red onion, cut into chunks
- Salt and black pepper to the taste
- 2 tablespoons Dijon mustard
- 2 and ½ tablespoons Worcestershire sauce
- ¼ cup tamari sauce
- ¼ cup lemon juice
- ½ cup olive oil

Directions:

1. In a bowl, mix Worcestershire sauce with salt, pepper, garlic, mustard, tamari, lemon juice and oil and whisk very well.
2. Add beef, bell peppers and onion chunks to this mix, toss to coat and leave aside for a few minutes.
3. Arrange bell pepper, meat cubes and onion chunks on skewers alternating colors, place them on your preheated grill over medium high heat, cook for 5 minutes on each side, transfer to a platter and serve as a summer keto appetizer.

Enjoy!

Nutrition: calories 246, fat 12, fiber 1, carbs 4, protein 26

Simple Zucchini Rolls

You've got to try this simple and very tasty appetizer as soon as possible!

Preparation time: 10 minutes

Cooking time: 5 minutes

Servings: 24

Ingredients:

- 2 tablespoons olive oil
- 3 zucchinis, thinly sliced
- 24 basil leaves
- 2 tablespoons mint, chopped
- 1 and 1/3 cup ricotta cheese
- Salt and black pepper to the taste
- ¼ cup basil, chopped
- Tomato sauce for serving

Directions:

1. Brush zucchini slices with the olive oil, season with salt and pepper on both sides, place them on preheated grill over medium heat, cook them for 2 minutes, flip and cook for another 2 minutes.

2. Place zucchini slices on a plate and leave aside for now.
3. In a bowl, mix ricotta with chopped basil, mint, salt and pepper and stir well.
4. Spread this over zucchini slices, divide whole basil leaves as well, roll and serve as an appetizer with some tomato sauce on the side.

Enjoy!

Nutrition: calories 40, fat 3, fiber 0.3, carbs 1, protein 2

Simple Green Crackers

These are real fun to make and they taste amazing!

Preparation time: 10 minutes

Cooking time: 24 hours

Servings: 6

Ingredients:

- 2 cups flax seed, ground
- 2 cups flax seed, soaked overnight and drained
- 4 bunches kale, chopped
- 1 bunch basil, chopped
- ½ bunch celery, chopped
- 4 garlic cloves, minced
- 1/3 cup olive oil

Directions:

1. In your food processor mix ground flaxseed with celery, kale, basil and garlic and blend well.
2. Add oil and soaked flaxseed and blend again.
3. Spread this on a tray, cut into medium crackers, introduce in your dehydrator and dry for 24 hours at 115 degrees F, turning them halfway.

4. Arrange them on a platter and serve.

Enjoy!

Nutrition: calories 100, fat 1, fiber 2, carbs 1, protein 4

Cheese And Pesto Terrine

This looks so amazing and it tastes great!

Preparation time: 30 minutes

Cooking time: 0 minutes

Servings: 10

Ingredients:

- ½ cup heavy cream
- 10 ounces goat cheese, crumbled
- 3 tablespoons basil pesto
- Salt and black pepper to the taste
- 5 sun-dried tomatoes, chopped
- ¼ cup pine nuts, toasted and chopped
- 1 tablespoons pine nuts, toasted and chopped

Directions:

1. In a bowl, mix goat cheese with the heavy cream, salt and pepper and stir using your mixer.
2. Spoon half of this mix into a lined bowl and spread.
3. Add pesto on top and also spread.
4. Add another layer of cheese, then add sun dried tomatoes and ¼ cup pine nuts.

5. Spread one last layer of cheese and top with 1 tablespoon pine nuts.
6. Keep in the fridge for a while, turn upside down on a plate and serve.

Enjoy!

Nutrition: calories 240, fat 12, fiber 3, carbs 5, protein 12

Avocado Salsa

You will make this over and over again! That's how tasty it is!

Preparation time: 10 minutes

Cooking time: 0 minutes

Servings: 4

Ingredients:

- 1 small red onion, chopped
- 2 avocados, pitted, peeled and chopped
- 3 jalapeno pepper, chopped
- Salt and black pepper to the taste
- 2 tablespoons cumin powder
- 2 tablespoons lime juice
- ½ tomato, chopped

Directions:

1. In a bowl, mix onion with avocados, peppers, salt, black pepper, cumin, lime juice and tomato pieces and stir well.
2. Transfer this to a bowl and serve with toasted baguette slices as a keto appetizer.

Enjoy!

Nutrition: calories 120, fat 2, fiber 2, carbs 0.4, protein 4

Tasty Egg Chips

Do you want to impress everyone? Then, try these chips!

Preparation time: 5 minutes

Cooking time: 10 minutes

Servings: 2

Ingredients:

- ½ tablespoon water
- 2 tablespoons parmesan, shredded
- 4 eggs whites
- Salt and black pepper to the taste

Directions:

1. In a bowl, mix egg whites with salt, pepper and water and whisk well.
2. Spoon this into a muffin pan, sprinkle cheese on top, introduce in the oven at 400 degrees F and bake for 15 minutes.
3. Transfer egg white chips to a platter and serve with a keto dip on the side.

Enjoy!

Nutrition: calories 120, fat 2, fiber 1, carbs 2, protein 7

Chili Lime Chips

These crackers will impress you with their amazing taste!

Preparation time: 10 minutes

Cooking time: 20 minutes

Servings: 4

Ingredients:

- 1 cup almond flour
- Salt and black pepper to the taste
- 1 and ½ teaspoons lime zest
- 1 teaspoon lime juice
- 1 egg

Directions:

1. In a bowl, mix almond flour with lime zest, lime juice and salt and stir.
2. Add egg and whisk well again.
3. Divide this into 4 parts, roll each into a ball and then spread well using a rolling pin.
4. Cut each into 6 triangles, place them all on a lined baking sheet, introduce in the oven at 350 degrees F and bake for 20 minutes.

Enjoy!

Nutrition: calories 90, fat 1, fiber 1, carbs 0.6, protein 3

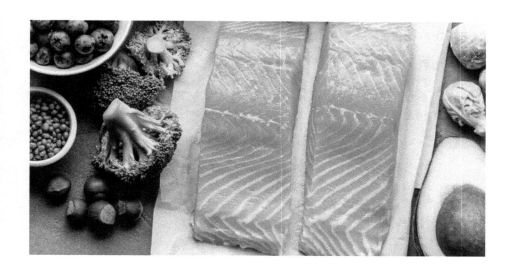

Artichoke Dip

It's so rich and flavored!

Preparation time: 10 minutes

Cooking time: 15 minutes

Servings: 16

Ingredients:

- ¼ cup sour cream
- ¼ cup heavy cream
- ¼ cup mayonnaise
- ¼ cup shallot, chopped
- 1 tablespoon olive oil
- 2 garlic cloves, minced
- 4 ounces cream cheese
- ½ cup parmesan cheese, grated
- 1 cup mozzarella cheese, shredded
- 4 ounces feta cheese, crumbled
- 1 tablespoon balsamic vinegar
- 28 ounces canned artichoke hearts, chopped
- Salt and black pepper to the taste
- 10 ounces spinach, chopped

Directions:

1. Heat up a pan with the oil over medium heat, add shallot and garlic, stir and cook for 3 minutes.
2. Add heavy cream and cream cheese and stir.
3. Also add sour cream, parmesan, mayo, feta cheese and mozzarella cheese, stir and reduce heat.
4. Add artichoke, spinach, salt, pepper and vinegar, stir well, take off heat and transfer to a bowl.
5. Serve as a tasty keto dip.

Enjoy!

Nutrition: calories 144, fat 12, fiber 2, carbs 5, protein 5

Ketogenic Fish And Seafood Recipes

Special Fish Pie

This is really creamy and rich!

Preparation time: 10 minutes

Cooking time: 1 hour and 10 minutes

Servings: 6

Ingredients:

- 1 red onion, chopped
- 2 salmon fillets, skinless and cut into medium pieces
- 2 mackerel fillets, skinless and cut into medium pieces
- 3 haddock fillets and cut into medium pieces
- 2 bay leaves
- ¼ cup ghee+ 2 tablespoons ghee
- 1 cauliflower head, florets separated
- 4 eggs
- 4 cloves
- 1 cup whipping cream
- ½ cup water
- A pinch of nutmeg, ground
- 1 teaspoon Dijon mustard
- 1 cup cheddar cheese, shredded+ ½ cup cheddar cheese, shredded
- Some chopped parsley

39

- Salt and black pepper to the taste
- 4 tablespoons chives, chopped

Directions:

1. Put some water in a pan, add some salt, bring to a boil over medium heat, add eggs, , cook them for 10 minutes, take off heat, drain, leave them to cool down, peel and cut them into quarters.
2. Put water in another pot, bring to a boil, add cauliflower florets, cook for 10 minutes, drain them, transfer to your blender, add ¼ cup ghee, pulse well and transfer to a bowl.
3. Put cream and ½ cup water in a pan, add fish, toss to coat and heat up over medium heat.
4. Add onion, cloves and bay leaves, bring to a boil, reduce heat and simmer for 10 minutes.
5. Take off heat, transfer fish to a baking dish and leave aside.
6. return pan with fish sauce to heat, add nutmeg, stir and cook for 5 minutes.
7. Take off heat, discard cloves and bay leaves, add 1 cup cheddar cheese and 2 tablespoons ghee and stir well.
8. Place egg quarters on top of the fish in the baking dish.
9. Add cream and cheese sauce over them, top with cauliflower mash, sprinkle the rest of the cheddar cheese, chives and parsley, introduce in the oven at 400 degrees F for 30 minutes.

10. Leave the pie to cool down a bit before slicing and serving.

Enjoy!

Nutrition: calories 300, fat 45, fiber 3, carbs 5, protein 26

Tasty Baked Fish

It's an easy keto dish for you to enjoy tonight for dinner!

Preparation time: 10 minutes

Cooking time: 30 minutes

Servings: 4

Ingredients:

- 1 pound haddock
- 3 teaspoons water
- 2 tablespoons lemon juice
- Salt and black pepper to the taste
- 2 tablespoons mayonnaise
- 1 teaspoon dill weed
- Cooking spray
- A pinch of old bay seasoning

Directions:

1. Spray a baking dish with some cooking oil.
2. Add lemon juice, water and fish and toss to coat a bit.
3. Add salt, pepper, old bay seasoning and dill weed and toss again.
4. Add mayo and spread well.

5. Introduce in the oven at 350 degrees F and bake for 30 minutes.

6. Divide between plates and serve.

Enjoy!

Nutrition: calories 104, fat 12, fiber 1, carbs 0.5, protein 20

Amazing Tilapia

This great dish is perfect for a special evening!

Preparation time: 10 minutes

Cooking time: 10 minutes

Servings: 4

Ingredients:

- 4 tilapia fillets, boneless
- Salt and black pepper to the taste
- ½ cup parmesan, grated
- 4 tablespoons mayonnaise
- ¼ teaspoon basil, dried
- ¼ teaspoon garlic powder
- 2 tablespoons lemon juice
- ¼ cup ghee
- Cooking spray
- A pinch of onion powder

Directions:

1. Spray a baking sheet with cooking spray, place tilapia on it, season with salt and pepper, introduce in preheated broiler and cook for 3 minutes.

2. Turn fish on the other side and broil for 3 minutes more.
3. In a bowl, mix parmesan with mayo, basil, garlic, lemon juice, onion powder and ghee and stir well.
4. Add fish to this mix, toss to coat well, place on baking sheet again and broil for 3 minutes more.
5. Transfer to plates and serve.

Enjoy!

Nutrition: calories 175, fat 10, fiber 0, carbs 2, protein 17

Amazing Trout And Special Sauce

You just have to try this wonderful combination! This keto dish is great!

Preparation time: 10 minutes

Cooking time: 10 minutes

Servings: 1

Ingredients:

- 1 big trout fillet
- Salt and black pepper to the taste
- 1 tablespoon olive oil
- 1 tablespoon ghee
- Zest and juice from 1 orange
- A handful parsley, chopped
- ½ cup pecans, chopped

Directions:

1. Heat up a pan with the oil over medium high heat, add the fish fillet, season with salt and pepper, cook for 4 minutes on each side, transfer to a plate and keep warm for now.

2. Heat up the same pan with the ghee over medium heat, add pecans, stir and toast for 1 minutes.

3. Add orange juice and zest, some salt and pepper and chopped parsley, stir, cook for 1 minute and pour over fish fillet.

4. Serve right away.

Enjoy!

Nutrition: calories 200, fat 10, fiber 2, carbs 1, protein 14

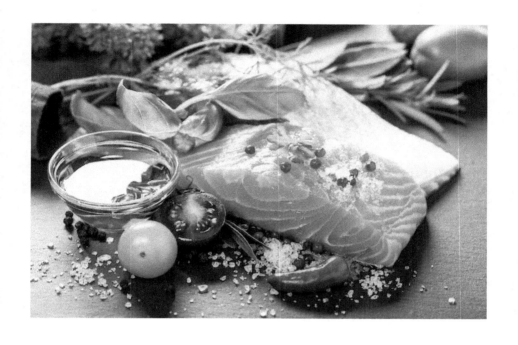

Wonderful Trout And Ghee Sauce

The fish goes so well with the sauce! You have to try today!

Preparation time: 10 minutes

Cooking time: 10 minutes

Servings: 4

Ingredients:

- 4 trout fillets
- Salt and black pepper to the taste
- 3 teaspoons lemon zest, grated
- 3 tablespoons chives, chopped
- 6 tablespoons ghee
- 2 tablespoons olive oil
- 2 teaspoons lemon juice

Directions:

1. Season trout with salt and pepper, drizzle the olive oil and massage a bit.
2. Heat up your kitchen grill over medium high heat, add fish fillets, cook for 4 minutes, flip and cook for 4 minutes more.

3. Meanwhile, heat up a pan with the ghee over medium heat, add salt, pepper, chives, lemon juice and zest and stir well.
4. Divide fish fillets on plates, drizzle the ghee sauce over them and serve.

Enjoy!

Nutrition: calories 320, fat 12, fiber 1, carbs 2, protein 24

Roasted Salmon

Feel free to serve this for a special occasion!

Preparation time: 10 minutes

Cooking time: 12 minutes

Servings: 4

Ingredients:

- 2 tablespoons ghee, soft
- 1 and ¼ pound salmon fillet
- 2 ounces Kimchi, finely chopped
- Salt and black pepper to the taste

Directions:

1. In your food processor, mix ghee with Kimchi and blend well.
2. Rub salmon with salt, pepper and Kimchi mix and place into a baking dish.
3. Introduce in the oven at 425 degrees F and bake for 15 minutes.
4. Divide between plates and serve with a side salad.

Enjoy!

Nutrition: calories 200, fat 12, fiber 0, carbs 3, protein 21

Delicious Salmon Meatballs

Combine these tasty salmon meatballs with a Dijon sauce and enjoy!

Preparation time: 10 minutes

Cooking time: 30 minutes

Servings: 4

Ingredients:

- 2 tablespoons ghee
- 2 garlic cloves, minced
- 1/3 cup onion, chopped
- 1 pound wild salmon, boneless and minced
- ¼ cup chives, chopped
- 1 egg
- 2 tablespoons Dijon mustard
- 1 tablespoon coconut flour
- Salt and black pepper to the taste

For the sauce:

- 4 garlic cloves, minced
- 2 tablespoons ghee
- 2 tablespoons Dijon mustard
- Juice and zest of 1 lemon

- 2 cups coconut cream
- 2 tablespoons chives, chopped

Directions:

1. Heat up a pan with 2 tablespoons ghee over medium heat, add onion and 2 garlic cloves, stir, cook for 3 minutes and transfer to a bowl.
2. In another bowl, mix onion and garlic with salmon, chives, coconut flour, salt, pepper, 2 tablespoons mustard and egg and stir well.
3. Shape meatballs from the salmon mix, place on a baking sheet, introduce in the oven at 350 degrees F and bake for 25 minutes.
4. Meanwhile, heat up a pan with 2 tablespoons ghee over medium heat, add 4 garlic cloves, stir and cook for 1 minute.
5. Add coconut cream, 2 tablespoons Dijon mustard, lemon juice and zest and chives, stir and cook for 3 minutes.
6. Take salmon meatballs out of the oven, drop them into the Dijon sauce, toss, cook for 1 minute and take off heat.
7. Divide into bowls and serve.

Enjoy!

Nutrition: calories 171, fat 5, fiber 1, carbs 6, protein 23

Salmon With Caper Sauce

This dish is wonderful and very simple to make!

Preparation time: 10 minutes

Cooking time: 20 minutes

Servings: 3

Ingredients:

- 3 salmon fillets
- Salt and black pepper to the taste
- 1 tablespoon olive oil
- 1 tablespoon Italian seasoning
- 2 tablespoons capers
- 3 tablespoons lemon juice
- 4 garlic cloves, minced
- 2 tablespoons ghee

Directions:

1. Heat up a pan with the olive oil over medium heat, add fish fillets skin side up, season them with salt, pepper and Italian seasoning, cook for 2 minutes, flip and cook for 2 more minutes, take off heat, cover pan and leave aside for 15 minutes.

2. Transfer fish to a plate and leave them aside.
3. Heat up the same pan over medium heat, add capers, lemon juice and garlic, stir and cook for 2 minutes.
4. Take the pan off the heat, add ghee and stir very well.
5. Return fish to pan and toss to coat with the sauce.
6. Divide between plates and serve.

Enjoy!

Nutrition: calories 245, fat 12, fiber 1, carbs 3, protein 23

Simple Grilled Oysters

These are so juicy and delicious!

Preparation time: 10 minutes

Cooking time: 10 minutes

Servings: 3

Ingredients:

- 6 big oysters, shucked
- 3 garlic cloves, minced
- 1 lemon cut in wedges
- 1 tablespoon parsley
- A pinch of sweet paprika
- 2 tablespoons melted ghee

Directions:

1. Top each oyster with melted ghee, parsley, paprika and ghee.
2. Place them on preheated grill over medium high heat and cook for 8 minutes.
3. Serve them with lemon wedges on the side.

Enjoy!

Nutrition: calories 60, fat 1, fiber 0, carbs 0.6, protein 1

Baked Halibut

This is a delicious fish and if you choose to make it this way you will really end up loving it!

Preparation time: 10 minutes

Cooking time: 10 minutes

Servings: 4

Ingredients:

- ½ cup parmesan, grated
- ¼ cup ghee
- ¼ cup mayonnaise
- 2 tablespoons green onions, chopped
- 6 garlic cloves, minced
- A dash of Tabasco sauce
- 4 halibut fillets
- Salt and black pepper to the taste
- Juice of ½ lemon

Directions:

1. Season halibut with salt, pepper and some of the lemon juice, place in a baking dish and cook in the oven at 450 degrees F for 6 minutes.

61

2. Meanwhile, heat up a pan with the ghee over medium heat, add parmesan, mayo, green onions, Tabasco sauce, garlic and the rest of the lemon juice and stir well.
3. Take fish out of the oven, drizzle parmesan sauce all over, turn oven to broil and broil your fish for 3 minutes.
4. Divide between plates and serve.

Enjoy!

Nutrition: calories 240, fat 12, fiber 1, carbs 5, protein 23

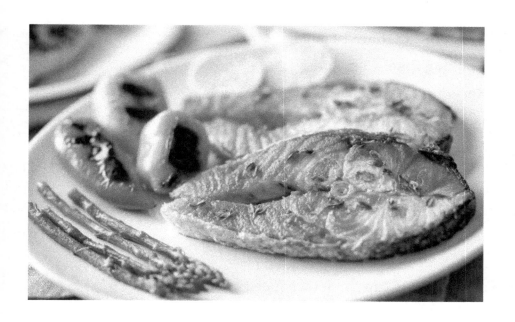

Crusted Salmon

The crust is wonderful!

Preparation time: 10 minutes

Cooking time: 15 minutes

Servings: 4

Ingredients:

- 3 garlic cloves, minced
- 2 pounds salmon fillet
- Salt and black pepper to the taste
- ½ cup parmesan, grated
- ¼ cup parsley, chopped

Directions:

1. Place salmon on a lined baking sheet, season with salt and pepper, cover with a parchment paper, introduce in the oven at 425 degrees F and bake for 10 minutes.
2. Take fish out of the oven, sprinkle parmesan, parsley and garlic over fish, introduce in the oven again and cook for 5 minutes more.
3. Divide between plates and serve.

Enjoy!

Nutrition: calories 240, fat 12, fiber 1, carbs 0.6, protein 25

Sour Cream Salmon

It's perfect keto dish for a weekend meal!

Preparation time: 10 minutes

Cooking time: 15 minutes

Servings: 4

Ingredients:

- 4 salmon fillets
- A drizzle of olive oil
- Salt and black pepper to the taste
- 1/3 cup parmesan, grated
- 1 and ½ teaspoon mustard
- ½ cup sour cream

Directions:

1. Place salmon on a lined baking sheet, season with salt and pepper and drizzle the oil.
2. In a bowl, mix sour cream with parmesan, mustard, salt and pepper and stir well.
3. Spoon this sour cream mix over salmon, introduce in the oven at 350 degrees F and bake for 15 minutes.
4. Divide between plates and serve.

Enjoy!

Nutrition: calories 200, fat 6, fiber 1, carbs 4, protein 20

Grilled Salmon

This grilled salmon must be served with an avocado salsa!

Preparation time: 30 minutes

Cooking time: 10 minutes

Servings: 4

Ingredients:

- 4 salmon fillets
- 1 tablespoon olive oil
- Salt and black pepper to the taste
- 1 teaspoon cumin, ground
- 1 teaspoon sweet paprika
- ½ teaspoon ancho chili powder
- 1 teaspoon onion powder

For the salsa:

- 1 small red onion, chopped
- 1 avocado, pitted, peeled and chopped
- 2 tablespoons cilantro, chopped
- Juice from 2 limes
- Salt and black pepper to the taste

Directions:

1. In a bowl, mix salt, pepper, chili powder, onion powder, paprika and cumin.
2. Rub salmon with this mix, drizzle the oil and rub again and cook on preheated grill for 4 minutes on each side.
3. Meanwhile, in a bowl, mix avocado with red onion, salt, pepper, cilantro and lime juice and stir.
4. Divide salmon between plates and top each fillet with avocado salsa.

Enjoy!

Nutrition: calories 300, fat 14, fiber 4, carbs 5, protein 20

Tasty Tuna Cakes

You just have to make these keto cakes for your family tonight!

Preparation time: 10 minutes

Cooking time: 10 minutes

Servings: 12

Ingredients:

- 15 ounces canned tuna, drain well and flaked
- 3 eggs
- ½ teaspoon dill, dried
- 1 teaspoon parsley, dried
- ½ cup red onion, chopped
- 1 teaspoon garlic powder
- Salt and black pepper to the taste
- Oil for frying

Directions:

1. In a bowl, mix tuna with salt, pepper, dill, parsley, onion, garlic powder and eggs and stir well.
2. Shape your cakes and place on a plate.
3. Heat up a pan with some oil over medium high heat, add tuna cakes, cook for 5 minutes on each side.

4. Divide between plates and serve.

Enjoy!

Nutrition: calories 140, fat 2, fiber 1, carbs 0.6, protein 6

Very Tasty Cod

Today, we recommend you to try a keto cod dish!

Preparation time: 10 minutes

Cooking time: 20 minutes

Servings: 4

Ingredients:

- 1 pound cod, cut into medium pieces
- Salt and black pepper to the taste
- 2 green onions, chopped
- 3 garlic cloves, minced
- 3 tablespoons soy sauce
- 1 cup fish stock
- 1 tablespoons balsamic vinegar
- 1 tablespoon ginger, grated
- ½ teaspoon chili pepper, crushed

Directions:

1. Heat up a pan over medium high heat, add fish pieces and brown it a few minutes on each side.

2. Add garlic, green onions, salt, pepper, soy sauce, fish stock, vinegar, chili pepper and ginger, stir, cover, reduce heat and cook for 20 minutes.
3. Divide between plates and serve.

Enjoy!

Nutrition: calories 154, fat 3, fiber 0.5, carbs 4, protein 24

Tasty Sea Bass With Capers

It's a very tasty and easy dish to make at home when you are on a keto diet!

Preparation time: 10 minutes

Cooking time: 15 minutes

Servings: 4

Ingredients:

- 1 lemon, sliced
- 1 pound sea bass fillet
- 2 tablespoons capers
- 2 tablespoons dill
- Salt and black pepper to the taste

Directions:

1. Put sea bass fillet into a baking dish, season with salt and pepper, add capers, dill and lemon slices on top.
2. Introduce in the oven at 350 degrees F and bake for 15 minutes.
3. Divide between plates and serve.

Enjoy!

Nutrition: calories 150, fat 3, fiber 2, carbs 0.7, protein 5

Cod With Arugula

It's an excellent keto meal that will be ready to serve in no time!

Preparation time: 10 minutes

Cooking time: 20 minutes

Servings: 2

Ingredients:

- 2 cod fillets
- 1 tablespoon olive oil
- Salt and black pepper to the taste
- Juice of 1 lemon
- 3 cup arugula
- ½ cup black olives, pitted and sliced
- 2 tablespoons capers
- 1 garlic clove, chopped

Directions:

1. Arrange fish fillets in a heatproof dish, season with salt, pepper, drizzle the oil and lemon juice, toss to coat, introduce in the oven at 450 degrees F and bake for 20 minutes.

2. In your food processor, mix arugula with salt, pepper, capers, olives and garlic and blend a bit.

3. Arrange fish on plates, top with arugula tapenade and serve.

Enjoy!

Nutrition: calories 240, fat 5, fiber 3, carbs 3, protein 10

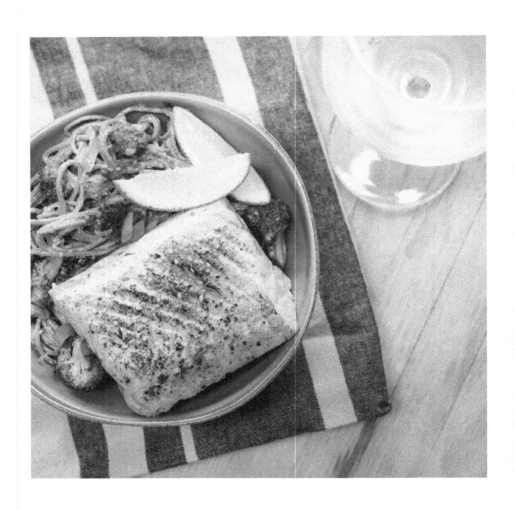

Baked Halibut And Veggies

You are going to love this great keto idea!

Preparation time: 10 minutes

Cooking time: 35 minutes

Servings: 2

Ingredients:

- 1 red bell pepper, roughly chopped
- 1 yellow bell pepper, roughly chopped
- 1 teaspoon balsamic vinegar
- 1 tablespoon olive oil
- 2 halibut fillets
- 2 cups baby spinach
- Salt and black pepper to the taste
- 1 teaspoon cumin

Directions:

1. In a bowl, mix bell peppers with salt, pepper, half of the oil and the vinegar, toss to coat well and transfer to a baking dish.
2. Introduce in the oven at 400 degrees F and bake for 20 minutes.

3. Heat up a pan with the rest of the oil over medium heat, add fish, season with salt, pepper and cumin and brown on all sides.
4. Take the baking dish out of the oven, add spinach, stir gently and divide the whole mix between plates.
5. Add fish on the side, sprinkle some more salt and pepper and serve.

Enjoy!

Nutrition: calories 230, fat 12, fiber 1, carbs 4, protein 9

Tasty Fish Curry

Have you ever tried a Ketogenic curry? Then you should really pay attention next!

Preparation time: 10 minutes

Cooking time: 25 minutes

Servings: 4

Ingredients:

- 4 white fish fillets
- ½ teaspoon mustard seeds
- Salt and black pepper to the taste
- 2 green chilies, chopped
- 1 teaspoon ginger, grated
- 1 teaspoon curry powder
- ¼ teaspoon cumin, ground
- 4 tablespoons coconut oil
- 1 small red onion, chopped
- 1 inch turmeric root, grated
- ¼ cup cilantro
- 1 and ½ cups coconut cream
- 3 garlic cloves, minced

Directions:

1. Heat up a pot with half of the coconut oil over medium heat, add mustard seeds and cook for 2 minutes.
2. Add ginger, onion and garlic, stir and cook for 5 minutes.
3. Add turmeric, curry powder, chilies and cumin, stir and cook for 5 minutes more.
4. Add coconut milk, salt and pepper, stir, bring to a boil and cook for 15 minutes.
5. Heat up another pan with the rest of the oil over medium heat, add fish, stir and cook for 3 minutes.
6. Add this to the curry sauce, stir and cook for 5 minutes more.
7. Add cilantro, stir, divide into bowls and serve.

Enjoy!

Nutrition: calories 500, fat 34, fiber 7, carbs 6, protein 44

Delicious Shrimp

It's an easy and tasty idea for dinner!

Preparation time: 10 minutes

Cooking time: 10 minutes

Servings: 4

Ingredients:

- 2 tablespoons olive oil
- 1 tablespoon ghee
- 1 pound shrimp, peeled and deveined
- 2 tablespoons lemon juice
- 2 tablespoons garlic, minced
- 1 tablespoon lemon zest
- Salt and black pepper to the taste

Directions:

1. Heat up a pan with the oil and the ghee over medium high heat, add shrimp and cook for 2 minutes.
2. Add garlic, stir and cook for 4 minutes more.
3. Add lemon juice, lemon zest, salt and pepper, stir, take off heat and serve.

Enjoy!

Nutrition: calories 149, fat 1, fiber 3, carbs 1, protein 6

Roasted Barramundi

This is an exceptional dish!

Preparation time: 10 minutes

Cooking time: 12 minutes

Servings: 4

Ingredients:

- 2 barramundi fillets
- 2 teaspoon olive oil
- 2 teaspoons Italian seasoning
- ¼ cup green olives, pitted and chopped
- ¼ cup cherry tomatoes, chopped
- ¼ cup black olives, chopped
- 1 tablespoon lemon zest
- 2 tablespoons lemon zest
- Salt and black pepper to the taste
- 2 tablespoons parsley, chopped
- 1 tablespoon olive oil

Directions:

1. Rub fish with salt, pepper, Italian seasoning and 2 teaspoons olive oil, transfer to a baking dish and leave aside for now.
2. Meanwhile, in a bowl, mix tomatoes with all the olives, salt, pepper, lemon zest and lemon juice, parsley and 1 tablespoon olive oil and toss everything well.
3. Introduce fish in the oven at 400 degrees F and bake for 12 minutes.
4. Divide fish on plates, top with tomato relish and serve.

Enjoy!

Nutrition: calories 150, fat 4, fiber 2, carbs 1, protein 10

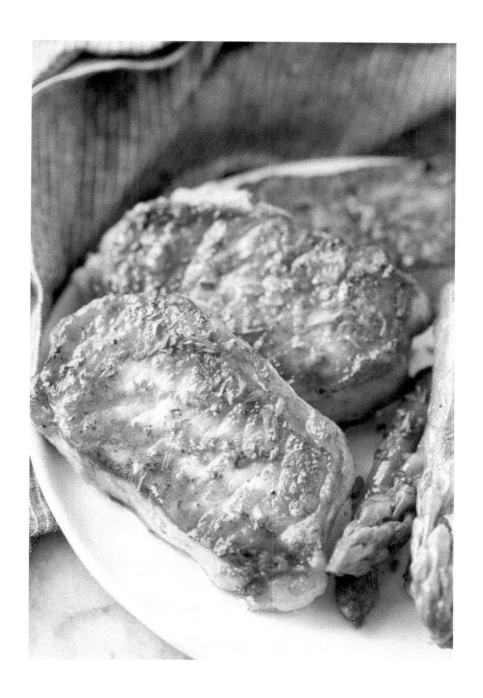

Sardines Salad

It's a rich and nutritious winter salad you have to try soon!

Preparation time: 10 minutes

Cooking time: 0 minutes

Servings: 1

Ingredients:

- 5 ounces canned sardines in oil
- 1 tablespoons lemon juice
- 1 small cucumber, chopped
- ½ tablespoon mustard
- Salt and black pepper to the taste

Directions:

1. Drain sardines, put them in a bowl and mash using a fork.
2. Add salt, pepper, cucumber, lemon juice and mustard, stir well and serve cold.

Enjoy!

Nutrition: calories 200, fat 20, fiber 1, carbs 0, protein 20

Italian Clams Delight

It's a special Italian delight! Serve this amazing dish to your family!

Preparation time: 10 minutes

Cooking time: 10 minutes

Servings: 6

Ingredients:

- ½ cup ghee
- 36 clams, scrubbed
- 1 teaspoon red pepper flakes, crushed
- 1 teaspoon parsley, chopped
- 5 garlic cloves, minced
- 1 tablespoon oregano, dried
- 2 cups white wine

Directions:

1. Heat up a pan with the ghee over medium heat, add garlic, stir and cook for 1 minute.
2. Add parsley, oregano, wine and pepper flakes and stir well.
3. Add clams, stir, cover and cook for 10 minutes.

4. Discard unopened clams, ladle clams and their mix into bowls and serve.

Enjoy!

Nutrition: calories 224, fat 15, fiber 2, carbs 3, protein 4

Orange Glazed Salmon

You must try this soon! It's a delicious keto fish recipe!

Preparation time: 10 minutes

Cooking time: 10 minutes

Servings: 2

Ingredients:

- 2 lemons, sliced
- 1 pound wild salmon, skinless and cubed
- ¼ cup balsamic vinegar
- ¼ cup red orange juice
- 1 teaspoon coconut oil
- 1/3 cup orange marmalade, no sugar added

Directions:

1. Heat up a pot over medium heat, add vinegar, orange juice and marmalade, stir well, bring to a simmer for 1 minute, reduce temperature, cook until it thickens a bit and take off heat.
2. Arrange salmon and lemon slices on skewers and brush them on one side with the orange glaze.

3. Brush your kitchen grill with coconut oil and heat up over medium heat.
4. Place salmon kebabs on grill with glazed side down and cook for 4 minutes.
5. Flip kebabs, brush them with the rest of the orange glaze and cook for 4 minutes more.
6. Serve right away.

Enjoy!

Nutrition: calories 160, fat 3, fiber 2, carbs 1, protein 8

Delicious Tuna And Chimichurri Sauce

Who wouldn't love this keto dish?

Preparation time: 10 minutes

Cooking time: 5 minutes

Servings: 4

Ingredients:

- ½ cup cilantro, chopped
- 1/3 cup olive oil
- 2 tablespoons olive oil
- 1 small red onion, chopped
- 3 tablespoon balsamic vinegar
- 2 tablespoons parsley, chopped
- 2 tablespoons basil, chopped
- 1 jalapeno pepper, chopped
- 1 pound sushi grade tuna steak
- Salt and black pepper to the taste
- 1 teaspoon red pepper flakes
- 1 teaspoon thyme, chopped
- A pinch of cayenne pepper
- 3 garlic cloves, minced

- 2 avocados, pitted, peeled and sliced
- 6 ounces baby arugula

Directions:

1. In a bowl, mix 1/3 cup oil with jalapeno, vinegar, onion, cilantro, basil, garlic, parsley, pepper flakes, thyme, cayenne, salt and pepper, whisk well and leave aside for now.
2. Heat up a pan with the rest of the oil over medium high heat, add tuna, season with salt and pepper, cook for 2 minutes on each side, transfer to a cutting board, leave aside to cool down a bit and slice.
3. Mix arugula with half of the chimichurri mix you've made and toss to coat.
4. Divide arugula on plates, top with tuna slices, drizzle the rest of the chimichurri sauce and serve with avocado slices on the side.

Enjoy!

Nutrition: calories 186, fat 3, fiber 1, carbs 4, protein 20

Salmon Bites And Chili Sauce

This is an amazing and super tasty combination!

Preparation time: 10 minutes

Cooking time: 15 minutes

Servings: 6

Ingredients:

- 1 and ¼ cups coconut, desiccated and unsweetened
- 1 pound salmon, cubed
- 1 egg
- Salt and black pepper
- 1 tablespoon water
- 1/3 cup coconut flour
- 3 tablespoons coconut oil

For the sauce:

- ¼ teaspoon agar agar
- 3 garlic cloves, chopped
- ¾ cup water
- 4 Thai red chilies, chopped
- ¼ cup balsamic vinegar
- ½ cup stevia

- A pinch of salt

Directions:

1. In a bowl, mix flour with salt and pepper and stir.
2. In another bowl, whisk egg and 1 tablespoon water.
3. Put the coconut in a third bowl.
4. Dip salmon cubes in flour, egg and then in coconut and place them on a plate.
5. Heat up a pan with the coconut oil over medium high heat, add salmon bites, cook for 3 minutes on each side and transfer them to paper towels.
6. Heat up a pan with ¾ cup water over high heat, sprinkle agar agar and bring to a boil.
7. Cook for 3 minutes and take off heat.
8. In your blender, mix garlic with chilies, vinegar, stevia and a pinch of salt and blend well.
9. Transfer this to a small pan and heat up over medium high heat.
10. Stir, add agar mix and cook for 3 minutes.
11. Serve your salmon bites with chili sauce on the side.

Enjoy!

Nutrition: calories 50, fat 2, fiber 0, carbs 4, protein 2

Irish Clams

It's an excellent idea for your dinner!

Preparation time: 10 minutes

Cooking time: 10 minutes

Servings: 4

Ingredients:

- 2 pounds clams, scrubbed
- 3 ounces pancetta
- 1 tablespoon olive oil
- 3 tablespoons ghee
- 2 garlic cloves, minced
- 1 bottle infused cider
- Salt and black pepper to the taste
- Juice of ½ lemon
- 1 small green apple, chopped
- 2 thyme springs, chopped

Directions:

1. Heat up a pan with the oil over medium high heat, add pancetta, brown for 3 minutes and reduce temperature to medium.

2. Add ghee, garlic, salt, pepper and shallot, stir and cook for 3 minutes.
3. Increase heat again, add cider, stir well and cook for 1 minute.
4. Add clams and thyme, cover pan and simmer for 5 minutes.
5. Discard unopened clams, add lemon juice and apple pieces, stir and divide into bowls.
6. Serve hot.

Enjoy!

Nutrition: calories 100, fat 2, fiber 1, carbs 1, protein 20

Seared Scallops And Roasted Grapes

A special occasion requires a special dish! Try these keto scallops!

Preparation time: 5 minutes

Cooking time: 10 minutes

Servings: 4

Ingredients:

- 1 pound scallops
- 3 tablespoons olive oil
- 1 shallot, chopped
- 3 garlic cloves, minced
- 2 cups spinach
- 1 cup chicken stock
- 1 romanesco lettuce head
- 1 and ½ cups red grapes, cut in halves
- ¼ cup walnuts, toasted and chopped
- 1 tablespoon ghee
- Salt and black pepper to the taste

Directions:

1. Put romanesco in your food processor, blend and transfer to a bowl.

99

2. Heat up a pan with 2 tablespoons oil over medium high heat, add shallot and garlic, stir and cook for 1 minute.
3. Add romanesco, spinach and 1 cup stock, stir, cook for 3 minutes, blend using an immersion blender and take off heat.
4. Heat up another pan with 1 tablespoon oil and the ghee over medium high heat, add scallops, season with salt and pepper, cook for 2 minutes, flip and sear for 1 minute more.
5. Divide romanesco mix on plates, add scallops on the side, top with walnuts and grapes and serve.

Enjoy!

Nutrition: calories 300, fat 12, fiber 2, carbs 6, protein 20

Oysters And Pico De Gallo

It's flavored and very delicious!

Preparation time: 10 minutes

Cooking time: 10 minutes

Servings: 6

Ingredients:

- 18 oysters, scrubbed
- A handful cilantro, chopped
- 2 tomatoes, chopped
- 1 jalapeno pepper, chopped
- ¼ cup red onion, finely chopped
- Salt and black pepper to the taste
- ½ cup Monterey Jack cheese, shredded
- 2 limes, cut into wedges
- Juice from 1 lime

Directions:

1. In a bowl, mix onion with jalapeno, cilantro, tomatoes, salt, pepper and lime juice and stir well.
2. Place oysters on preheated grill over medium high heat, cover grill and cook for 7 minutes until they open.

3. Transfer opened oysters to a heatproof dish and discard unopened ones.
4. Top oysters with cheese and introduce in preheated broiler for 1 minute.
5. Arrange oysters on a platter, top each with tomatoes mix you've made earlier and serve with lime wedges on the side.

Enjoy!

Nutrition: calories 70, fat 2, fiber 0, carbs 1, protein 1

Grilled Squid And Tasty Guacamole

The squid combines perfectly with the delicious guacamole!

Preparation time: 10 minutes

Cooking time: 10 minutes

Servings: 2

Ingredients:

- 2 medium squids, tentacles separated and tubes scored lengthwise
- A drizzle of olive oil
- Juice from 1 lime
- Salt and black pepper to the taste

For the guacamole:

- 2 avocados, pitted, peeled and chopped
- Some coriander springs, chopped
- 2 red chilies, chopped
- 1 tomato, chopped
- 1 red onion, chopped
- Juice from 2 limes

Directions:

1. Season squid and squid tentacles with salt, pepper, drizzle some olive oil and massage well.
2. Place on preheated grill over medium high heat score side down and cook for 2 minutes.
3. Flip and cook for 2 minutes more and transfer to a bowl.
4. Add juice from 1 lime, toss to coat and keep warm.
5. Put avocado in a bowl and mash using a fork.
6. Add coriander, chilies, tomato, onion and juice from 2 limes and stir well everything.
7. Divide squid on plates, top with guacamole and serve.

Enjoy!

Nutrition: calories 500, fat 43, fiber 6, carbs 7, protein 20

Shrimp And Cauliflower Delight

It looks good and it tastes amazing!

Preparation time: 10 minutes

Cooking time: 15 minutes

Servings: 2

Ingredients:

- 1 tablespoon ghee
- 1 cauliflower head, florets separated
- 1 pound shrimp, peeled and deveined
- ¼ cup coconut milk
- 8 ounces mushrooms, roughly chopped
- A pinch of red pepper flakes
- Salt and black pepper to the taste
- 2 garlic cloves, minced
- 4 bacon slices
- ½ cup beef stock
- 1 tablespoon parsley, finely chopped
- 1 tablespoon chives, chopped

Directions:

1. Heat up a pan over medium high heat, add bacon, cook until it's crispy, transfer to paper towels and leave aside.
2. Heat up another pan with 1 tablespoon bacon fat over medium high heat, add shrimp, cook for 2 minutes on each side and transfer to a bowl.
3. Heat up the pan again over medium heat, add mushrooms, stir and cook for 3-4 minutes.
4. Add garlic, pepper flakes, stir and cook for 1 minute.
5. Add beef stock, salt, pepper and return shrimp to pan as well.
6. Stir, cook until everything thickens a bit, take off heat and keep warm.
7. Meanwhile, put cauliflower in your food processor and mince it.
8. Place this into a heated pan over medium high heat, stir and cook for 5 minutes.
9. Add ghee and butter, stir and blend using an immersion blender.
10. Add salt and pepper to the taste, stir and divide into bowls.
11. Top with shrimp mix and serve with parsley and chives sprinkled all over.

Enjoy!

Nutrition: calories 245, fat 7, fiber 4, carbs 6, protein 20

Salmon Stuffed With Shrimp

It will soon become one of your favorite keto recipes!

Preparation time: 10 minutes

Cooking time: 25 minutes

Servings: 2

Ingredients:

- 2 salmon fillets
- A drizzle of olive oil
- 5 ounces tiger shrimp, peeled, deveined and chopped
- 6 mushrooms, chopped
- 3 green onions, chopped
- 2 cups spinach
- ¼ cup macadamia nuts, toasted and chopped
- Salt and black pepper to the taste
- A pinch of nutmeg
- ¼ cup mayonnaise

Directions:

1. Heat up a pan with the oil over medium high heat, add mushrooms, onions, salt and pepper, stir and cook for 4 minutes.

2. Add macadamia nuts, stir and cook for 2 minutes.
3. Add spinach, stir and cook for 1 minute.
4. Add shrimp, stir and cook for 1 minutes.
5. Take off heat, leave aside for a few minutes, add mayo and nutmeg and stir well.
6. Make an incision lengthwise in each salmon fillet, sprinkle salt and pepper, divide spinach and shrimp mix into incisions and place on a working surface.
7. Heat up a pan with a drizzle of oil over medium high heat, add stuffed salmon, skin side down, cook for 1 minutes, reduce temperature, cover pan and cook for 8 minutes.
8. Broil for 3 minutes, divide between plates and serve.

Enjoy!

Nutrition: calories 430, fat 30, fiber 3, carbs 7, protein 50

Mustard Glazed Salmon

This is one of our favorite keto salmon dishes! You will feel the same!

Preparation time: 10 minutes

Cooking time: 20 minutes

Servings: 1

Ingredients:

- 1 big salmon fillet
- Salt and black pepper to the taste
- 2 tablespoons mustard
- 1 tablespoon coconut oil
- 1 tablespoon maple extract

Directions:

1. In a bowl, mix maple extract with mustard and whisk well.
2. Season salmon with salt and pepper and brush salmon with half of the mustard mix
3. Heat up a pan with the oil over medium high heat, place salmon flesh side down and cook for 5 minutes.

4. Brush salmon with the rest of the mustard mix, transfer to a baking dish, introduce in the oven at 425 degrees F and bake for 15 minutes.
5. Serve with a tasty side salad.

Enjoy!

Nutrition: calories 240, fat 7, fiber 1, carbs 5, protein 23

Incredible Salmon Dish

You will make this over and over again!

Preparation time: 10 minutes

Cooking time: 15 minutes

Servings: 4

Ingredients:

- 3 cups ice water
- 2 teaspoons sriracha sauce
- 4 teaspoons stevia
- 3 scallions, chopped
- Salt and black pepper to the taste
- 2 teaspoons flaxseed oil
- 4 teaspoons apple cider vinegar
- 3 teaspoons avocado oil
- 4 medium salmon fillets
- 4 cups baby arugula
- 2 cups cabbage, finely chopped
- 1 and ½ teaspoon Jamaican jerk seasoning
- ¼ cup pepitas, toasted
- 2 cups watermelon radish, julienned

Directions:

1. Put ice water in a bowl, add scallions and leave aside.
2. In another bowl, mix sriracha sauce with stevia and stir well.
3. Transfer 2 teaspoons of this mix to a bowl and mix with half of the avocado oil, flaxseed oil, vinegar, salt and pepper and whisk well.
4. Sprinkle jerk seasoning over salmon, rub with sriracha and stevia mix and season with salt and pepper.
5. Heat up a pan with the rest of the avocado oil over medium high heat, add salmon, flesh side down, cook for 4 minutes, flip and cook for 4 minutes more and divide between plates.
6. In a bowl, mix radishes with cabbage and arugula.
7. Add salt, pepper, sriracha and vinegar mix and toss well.
8. Add this next to salmon fillets, drizzle the remaining sriracha and stevia sauce all over and top with pepitas and drained scallions.

Enjoy!

Nutrition: calories 160, fat 6, fiber 1, carbs 1, protein 12

Lightning Source UK Ltd.
Milton Keynes UK
UKHW020640060521
383241UK00015B/1144